PREGNANCY AND BIRTH CONTROL:
Your Family Planning Tips

Kelly Brown

Table of Contents

CHAPTER ONE
CHAPTER TWO
CHAPTER THREE
CHAPTER FOUR
CHAPTER FIVE
CHAPTER SIX

CHAPTER ONE

Introduction

One of life's most significant and transformational events is the road to parenting. While there will be many happy, exciting, and awe-inspiring moments along the way, there will also be plenty of difficult choices to make. This manual is intended to be your go-to companion whether you're a parent now, want to be one, or are just interested in learning about the complexities of reproductive health.

Two essential components of reproductive health that have a significant impact on both people and couples are pregnancy and birth control. They stand for the two opposing sides of a coin, one signifying the beginning of life and the other providing power and options over the time of that beginning. Both are very meaningful and highly personal.

We shall set off on a voyage of discovery and comprehension in the pages that follow. We'll explore the intricate workings of the female reproductive system, sort through the many birth control methods that are now accessible, and make choices about parenthood, wellness, and pregnancy.

This manual is your road map, whether you're looking to better understand your own body, choose contraception wisely, get ready for a safe pregnancy, or negotiate the challenging terrain of motherhood.

Our mission is to provide you with information, dispel common myths, and give you the resources you need to make decisions that are in line with your own needs, objectives, and circumstances.

Keep in mind that you are not traveling alone. Many have gone before you on this road, and many more will. We will jointly examine the marvels of human reproduction and the wide range of choices open to both individuals and couples in their search for a happy and healthy family life.

So let's start this path of understanding, empowerment, and decision-making. Greetings from the realm of conception and contraception, where information is your best friend.

CHAPTER TWO

The Female Reproductive System: The Basics.

A complex and extensive network of organs, the female reproductive system is in charge of creating eggs (ova), aiding fertilization, sustaining pregnancy, and delivering birth. The main elements are as follows:

Ovaries:
On either side of the lower abdomen are two ovaries.
The main female reproductive organs are the ovaries.
They create and store eggs (ova), as well as estrogen and progesterone, the female sex hormones.
ovaries' tubes
The ovaries and uterus are connected by these thin tubes.
They act as a conduit for the movement of eggs from the ovaries to the uterus.
Normally, sperm and eggs are fertilized in the fallopian tubes.

womb (uterus)
The uterus is a muscular, pear-shaped organ that is situated in the pelvic.

Its main job during pregnancy is to sustain and feed a fertilized egg.

Every month, the uterine lining becomes thicker in anticipation of a potential pregnancy; if one doesn't happen, it is shed throughout the menstrual cycle.

Cervix:

The lowest portion of the uterus that joins the vagina is known as the cervix.

In its role as a gatekeeper, it opens during menstruation to let menstrual blood through and mostly closes during pregnancy to safeguard the growing baby.

Vagina:

The muscular, tube-shaped vagina is the structure that connects the cervix to the external genitals.

It functions as a route for a baby to pass through during birthing and for menstrual blood to leave the body.

Outside Genitalia:

These include the clitoris, the vaginal entrance, and the labia (outer and inner "lips").

They function as the reproductive system's entrance and exit sites as well as a factor in sexual stimulation.

Periodic Cycle:

A natural, monthly process known as the menstrual cycle affects people with female reproductive systems. It entails a number of hormonal and physiological adjustments, mostly aimed at getting the body ready for a prospective pregnancy. The fundamental phases of the menstrual cycle are as follows:

Period (Days 1 through 5):

On the first day of menstruation, sometimes referred to as a period, the menstrual cycle starts. The uterine lining sheds during this phase and leaves the body via the vagina. It had grown thicker during the previous cycle in preparation for a prospective pregnancy.

Normal menstrual bleeding lasts 3 to 7 days.

Phase of the Follicle (Days 1–13):

Follicle-Stimulating Hormone (FSH) is released by the brain's pituitary gland at the same time as menstruation.

A number of small sacs called follicles, each carrying an immature egg (ova), are produced by the ovaries as a result of FSH stimulation.
Even while many follicles begin to form, usually only one develops and becomes the dominant follicle.
(Day 14) Ovulation
Ovulation is brought on by a spike in the luteinizing hormone (LH), which occurs in the middle of the menstrual cycle.

The mature egg is released from the ovary into the fallopian tube during ovulation.
Sexual activity at this period will increase the likelihood of pregnancy since it is the most fertile phase of the menstrual cycle.
Luteal Phase (15–28 Days):
The empty follicle develops into a structure known as the corpus luteum after ovulation.

Progesterone, a hormone produced by the corpus luteum, primes the uterine lining for prospective embryo implantation.

The corpus luteum continues to generate progesterone if pregnancy develops, supporting the early pregnancy.

The corpus luteum degenerates, progesterone levels fall, and the uterine lining starts to deteriorate if pregnancy does not take place, which starts menstruation.

Important Points:

Although it might vary from person to person, the average menstrual cycle lasts around 28 days.

Ovulation usually happens in the middle of the cycle, however this might change.

Menstrual cycle tracking may help people identify their fertile window and make plans for or avoid conception based on it.

The regularity and duration of menstrual periods may be influenced by a number of circumstances, including stress, sickness, and weight changes.

Although the major purpose of the menstrual cycle is reproductive, it also affects a person's general health and well-being.

The monthly cycle that the female reproductive system follows is known as the menstrual cycle. Although it might vary from person to person, it usually lasts for around 28 days.
Ovulation, which is the release of an egg from one of the ovaries, uterine lining thickening, and either menstruation, which is the shedding of the uterine lining in the absence of pregnancy, or preparation for pregnancy, are all parts of the menstrual cycle.

Hormonal Control:
Hormones, particularly estrogen and progesterone, control the female reproductive system.
These hormones regulate a number of menstrual cycle processes, including egg formation, uterine lining thickness and shedding, and many more.
For family planning, knowledge of fertility, and general reproductive health, it is essential to

understand the female reproductive system. A person's capacity to conceive, carry a pregnancy to term, and give birth depends heavily on it. Additionally, it affects a person's menstrual cycle and a variety of other sexual health issues.

Cycle Of Menstruation And Fertility

Fertility and the menstrual cycle are interrelated components of a person's reproductive health. Let's go more into these two ideas:

Periodic Cycle:
The menstrual cycle is a common, monthly process that people with female reproductive systems go through. Although it may vary, the average cycle lasts around 28 days. It has numerous crucial stages and is regulated by hormonal changes:
Menstruation: Also referred to as a period, menstruation is the first stage of the cycle. The uterine lining, which had grown thicker in the preceding cycle in anticipation of a prospective

pregnancy, is shed and evacuated from the body via the vagina during this phase.

The follicular phase is when menstruation occurs. Follicle-Stimulating Hormone (FSH), which is released by the pituitary gland in the brain, causes the ovaries to create several follicles, each of which contains an immature egg (ova). Even while multiple follicles begin to form, usually only one develops and becomes the dominant follicle.

Ovulation: Ovulation is brought on by an increase in the luteinizing hormone (LH), which occurs in the middle of the menstrual cycle. The developed egg is released from the ovary into the fallopian tube during ovulation, where it may be fertilized by sperm.
Luteal Phase: Following ovulation, the empty follicle develops into the corpus luteum, a structure. Progesterone, a hormone produced by the corpus luteum, primes the uterine lining for prospective embryo implantation. In the absence of pregnancy, the uterine lining starts to

deteriorate, the corpus luteum degenerates, progesterone levels fall, and menstruation begins, restarting the cycle.

Fertility:
The term "fertility" describes a person's capacity for sexual reproduction leading to conception and the birth of children. It stands for the ability to have a fruitful pregnancy. The ovulation phase of the menstrual cycle, which is the most fertile, is strongly connected to fertility. For a number of reasons, it is essential to understand fertility:

Family Planning: If a person or couple wants to become pregnant, knowing when ovulation happens might help them schedule their sexual activity to coincide with conception.
Understanding the fertile window can help you choose and use contraception to avoid conception when it is wanted.

Reproductive Health: Keeping track of the menstrual cycle might provide you important information about your general reproductive health. Cycle irregularities or ovulation problems may be signs of underlying health problems.

Fertility normally falls with age, and this reduction becomes more pronounced beyond the age of 35. Anyone thinking about becoming a parent later in life should be aware of this issue.
In conclusion, menstrual cycles and fertility are linked, with menstruation acting as a significant predictor of fertility. For family planning, managing reproductive health, and making educated choices about pregnancy and contraception, it is essential to comprehend both ideas.

CHAPTER THREE

Methods of Contraception

Contraception, often known as birth control methods, refers to a broad range of procedures and tactics used to avoid becoming pregnant by either preventing conception or interfering with the implantation of a fertilized egg. These techniques may be roughly divided into a number of types, each with its own mechanism and level of efficacy. Here is a thorough breakdown of the many birth control options:

Barrier Techniques:

Condoms: These are sheaths that cover the penis or line the vagina and are constructed of latex, polyurethane, or natural materials to stop sperm from fertilizing eggs. Additionally, condoms provide some STI (sexually transmitted illness) prevention.
A person puts a diaphragm or cervical cap into the vagina to cover the cervix and prevent sperm from reaching the uterus. They are used with spermicide to increase their potency.

Cervical Shield is a more recent barrier technique that uses a silicone cup to protect the cervix and spermicide within.

Hormonal Techniques

Birth control pills: These oral drugs suppress ovulation, thicken cervical mucus to block sperm, and change the uterine lining to lessen the likelihood of implantation. They often include a mix of estrogen and progestin or progestin-only.

Birth Control Patch:
 This is a tiny, adhesive patch that is applied to the skin and delivers hormones that are comparable to those found in birth control tablets.
A flexible, plastic birth control ring that is put into the vagina distributes hormones. Users take it off for one week during their menstrual cycle, after which it stays in place for three weeks.

Birth Control Shot (Depo-Provera): A progestin-only injectable given by a medical professional every three months.

Implants (Nexplanon): A little rod that may prevent pregnancy for up to three years after being implanted under the skin of the arm.

Intrauterine Devices (IUDs): A healthcare professional inserts these T-shaped devices into the uterus. They may be copper-based (ParaGard, for example) or hormonal (Mirena, Skyla, etc.) and provide long-term contraception.

Natural Techniques:

Monitoring cervical mucus, charting menstrual cycles, and measuring basal body temperature are all examples of fertility awareness-based methods (FAM), which are used to detect fertile days and prevent unprotected sexual activity.

The male partner withdraws the penis from the vagina before to ejaculation in the withdrawal (Pull-Out Method), although this technique is not very successful.

Permanent Techniques

A surgical treatment known as tubal ligation (female sterilization) involves blocking or sealing the fallopian tubes to stop eggs from entering the uterus.

Vasectomy (Male Sterilization): A surgical technique in which the vas deferens is severed or blocked to stop sperm from reaching the semen.

Rapid birth control:

These treatments, sometimes referred to as the "morning-after pill," may be used to lower the chance of conception after unprotected sexual activity. They might include inserting an IUD made of copper or hormones.

It's crucial to remember that no type of birth control is 100% effective, and that efficacy might change depending on use guidelines and individual circumstances. The best approach to use will depend on personal preferences, health factors, and contraceptive objectives. To examine choices and choose the best course of action for one's requirements and circumstances, it is essential to speak with a healthcare professional. In addition, barrier techniques like condoms provide defense against sexually transmitted diseases (STIs), which should be taken into account while planning sexual health.

Considerations for Method Selection

The best birth control technique should be chosen on a personal basis based on preferences, health factors, and contraceptive objectives. When selecting a birth control technique, keep the following things in mind:
Effectiveness: Take into account how successful the technique is in preventing pregnancy. Condoms and fertility awareness techniques have lower typical-use efficacy rates than hormone implants and intrauterine devices (IUDs), which are both very effective procedures.

Health and Medical History:
  Your decision may be influenced by your present health and medical history. For instance:

If you have a history of blood clots or certain medical issues, certain hormonal treatments may not be right for you.

Age and smoking may have an impact on how safe hormonal birth control is.
For people who cannot utilize hormonal therapies, copper-based IUDs might be a useful alternative.
Side Effects: The side effects of various birth control regimens might vary. Hormonal treatments may cause changes in some people's menstrual cycles, weight, mood, or libido. With your healthcare practitioner, go through any possible side effects.

Short-Term vs. Long-Term:
Take into account your future goals. IUDs and implants are two options if you desire a long-term contraceptive technique. The diaphragm, condoms, and birth control tablets are examples of short-term solutions.

Usefulness:

Consider how handy and pleasant an approach is for you. For instance:

It's important to take birth control tablets every day.

Although condoms are simple to use, they must always be used properly.

IUDs and implants are durable and need little upkeep.

Price:

The price of birth control varies. While certain treatments may be paid for by health insurance, others are paid for out-of-pocket. Choose a technique after taking your budget into account.

STI Protection: Barrier measures like condoms provide dual protection against both pregnancy and STIs if preventing sexually transmitted infections (STIs) is a concern.

Desire for Hormonal vs. Hormone-Free treatments: Hormonal treatments, such as hormonal IUDs and birth control tablets, include artificial hormones that alter the menstrual cycle. Consider non-hormonal techniques like copper

IUDs, condoms, or fertility awareness techniques if you want hormone-free choices.

Reversibility: Some procedures may be undone more quickly than others. Consider techniques that can be stopped without a significant loss of fertility if you want to have children soon, such as discontinuing birth control tablets.
Birth control techniques may have an effect on the menstrual period. Some techniques may induce irregular bleeding, while others may cause lighter or nonexistent periods. Consult your healthcare

practitioner about your choices.
Counseling and education: Make sure you understand exactly how to use your technique of choice. For greatest efficacy, many techniques need for the right technique.

Religious and Cultural views:
Your choice of contraception may be influenced by your cultural background and personal views.

With a healthcare professional who respects your views, talk about these issues.

It's important to keep in mind that there is no one-size-fits-all method of birth control, and what works best for one individual may not be the greatest option for another. It's crucial to speak with a healthcare professional who can provide you individualized advice based on your unique requirements and circumstances. Your chosen birth control method should continue to satisfy your requirements over time if there is open communication and frequent check-ins with your doctor.

Effects of Contraceptive Techniques

Although not everyone experiences them and the severity may vary from person to person, birth control techniques can have a number of negative effects. When selecting a birth control technique, it is crucial to go through possible adverse effects with a healthcare professional.

The following are some typical negative effects of various birth control methods:

Methods of hormonal birth control.
Pills for birth control.
Nausea, breast discomfort, changes in menstrual flow (lighter or heavier cycles), spotting in between periods, and mood swings are common side effects.
Weight changes, headaches, libido changes, and breakthrough bleeding are less common side effects.

(Transdermal Patch) Birth Control:
Skin irritation at the patch location, breast soreness, and side effects like those of birth control tablets are typical adverse effects.
Vaginal ring for birth control:
Vaginal discharge and adverse symptoms comparable to those of birth control tablets are typical side effects.

Vaccine for birth control (Depo-Provera):

Regular monthly flow, weight gain, and mood swings are common side effects.

Less frequent side effects include bone density decrease (especially with continued treatment).

Nexplanon implants

Menstrual irregularities, alterations in the menstrual cycle, migraines, and mood swings are typical side effects.

IUDs: Intrauterine devices

Hormonal IUDs (like Skyla and Mirena):

Regular bleeding, including spotting or periods not occurring, is a side effect that is typical with birth control implants.

IUD made of copper (ParaGard)

Menstrual cramps and more bleeding are typical side effects.

Birth Control Without Hormones

Barrier Techniques (Diaphragm, Condoms):

Allergic responses to latex (found in condoms), possible pain, or insertion challenges are common side effects.

IUD made of copper (ParaGard)
Menstrual cramps and more bleeding are typical side effects.

Natural Techniques:

Methods based on fertility awareness (FAM):
No overt side effects, but efficacy relies on precise monitoring and condom usage or abstinence during fertile days.

Permanent Techniques

Female Sterilization Through Tubal Ligation
Surgery risks and consequences, such as infection and postoperative discomfort, are common side effects.
(Male Sterilization) Vasectomy
Surgery risks and consequences, such as infection and postoperative discomfort, are common side effects.

It's essential to remember that many of the negative effects associated with hormonal birth control techniques are often minor and tend to subside as the body becomes used to the hormones. However, it's essential to speak with your healthcare physician if you suffer serious or persistent adverse effects. They may assist you in investigating alternate approaches or modifying your existing approach to reduce negative effects.

For individuals who would rather forego hormonal contraception, non-hormonal options are also offered, including copper IUDs and barrier techniques. Individual reactions to birth control techniques vary, thus selecting the best method should require a conversation with a healthcare professional to balance efficacy, side effects, and personal preferences.

CHAPTER FOUR

Pregnancy Preparation

Preconception wellness and health relate to the actions and routines that people or couples may follow prior to trying to conceive. Because it lays the groundwork for a good pregnancy and the wellbeing of both the mother and the child, it is a crucial stage in reproductive health. The following are significant elements of preconception wellness:

Consultation with Medical Professionals
Make an appointment for a preconception visit with a medical professional, especially one who specializes in obstetrics or reproductive health.
Talk to your doctor about your pregnancy intentions, health history, family history, and any underlying issues.

Taking Care of Chronic Conditions

Work with your healthcare professional to make sure any chronic health issues, such as diabetes, hypertension, or epilepsy, are properly controlled prior to conception.

To be sure they are safe to use during pregnancy, certain drugs may need to be altered or modified.

Vitamins for pregnancy and folic acid

Before conception, start taking a prenatal vitamin or folic acid supplement. A growing fetus has a lower chance of neural tube abnormalities if they consume enough folic acid. Start using these vitamins ideally a month or more before attempting pregnancy.

How to Reach a Healthy Weight:

Keep a healthy body weight before becoming pregnant. Conditions such as being underweight or overweight may have an impact on fertility and the health of a pregnancy.

To reach and maintain a healthy weight, strive for a balanced diet and consistent exercise.

Giving up drugs, alcohol, and smoking:
Avoid using recreational drugs, drinking, or smoking before becoming pregnant since they may damage the fetus and raise pregnancy risks.

Stress management and mental health:
High stress levels and untreated mental health issues may have an impact on a woman's ability to conceive and deliver a baby.
If necessary, use stress-reduction strategies like mindfulness, meditation, or therapy.

Vaccinations:
As certain infections that may be prevented by immunizations might be hazardous during pregnancy, be sure that your vaccinations are current.
If any extra shots are advised before conception, talk with your doctor about them.

Performing an infection check
Sexually transmitted infections (STIs) should be screened for since untreated infections might cause problems during pregnancy.

Before becoming pregnant, get the necessary therapy if you have a STI.

Limiting Exposure to Environmental Hazards and Toxins:
Reduce exposure to dangerous substances and environmental contaminants that may damage fertility and fetal development, such as lead or pesticides.

Choices for a Healthy Lifestyle:
Adopt a healthy lifestyle that consists of consistent exercise, a well-balanced food, and enough sleep.
Avoid consuming coffee in excess, and talk to your doctor about any dietary issues.

Recognizing the Menstrual Cycle:
The best days for conception may be found by monitoring your menstrual cycle and ovulation.
Goals for Family Planning are discussed:
Talk openly and honestly with your spouse about your family planning objectives, such as how many kids you want and when to have them.

Emotional and Financial Preparedness:
Examine your financial preparedness for motherhood, taking into account daycare and medical bills.
Think about how emotionally prepared you are for parenthood's demands.

The likelihood of a good pregnancy and healthy offspring may be increased by taking proactive measures to enhance your health and wellbeing before conception. For individualized advice and suggestions based on your unique health and family planning requirements, speak with a healthcare professional.

Timing and Awareness of Fertility

For people or couples who seek to conceive or prevent pregnancy, timing and fertility awareness are crucial aspects of family planning. These objectives may be successfully attained by knowing when fertility occurs throughout the menstrual cycle and how to monitor it. Key elements of timing and fertility awareness include:

Learning about the Menstrual Cycle:
Although it might vary, the menstrual cycle normally lasts around 28 days. Menstruation, the follicular phase, ovulation, and the luteal phase are among the stages that make up this cycle.

Ovulation:
The most fertile part of the menstrual cycle, ovulation is the release of a mature egg from the ovary.
Ovulation typically takes place 14 days before to the beginning of the subsequent menstrual period, in the middle of the menstrual cycle. However, this time might differ across people and cycles.
Monitoring ovulation

There are many ways to monitor ovulation:
1.Calculating fertile days using a calendar and previous menstrual cycles. This approach works

well for those with fairly regular cycles but is less precise.

2.Basal Body Temperature (BBT): Checking your body temperature each morning for a little increase that might be an ovulation sign.

3.Examining variations in cervical mucus consistency (which, on fertile days, becomes clear, slick, and stretchy).

4.Ovulation Predictor Kits (OPKs): These are at-home test kits that may identify an increase in luteinizing hormone (LH) before ovulation.

Numerous internet resources and applications for smartphones that monitor menstrual cycles and forecast fertile days are available.

Fertile Period

The time surrounding ovulation when conception is most likely to happen is known as the fertile window. Usually, it lasts a few days both before and after ovulation.

To increase their chances of becoming pregnant, couples who are trying to become pregnant should try to have sexual relations within the fertile window.

Fertility awareness as a method of birth control
Methods of fertility awareness may also be used to prevent conception via natural birth control. During the fertile window, couples may refrain from unprotected sexual contact.
It's crucial to remember that fertility awareness techniques need to be utilized appropriately and consistently tracked and aware in order to be successful.

Consistency and Regularity:
The regularity and consistency of menstrual cycles affect how well fertility awareness techniques work. Cycle irregularities might make monitoring more difficult.

Meeting with Experts:
Consider speaking with a healthcare professional or fertility expert if you are utilizing fertility awareness techniques for family planning. This will provide you advice and ensure that the approach you choose is in line with your objectives and physical well-being.

Backup techniques

To increase the success of their contraception, some couples decide to use barrier methods (like condoms) in addition to fertility awareness techniques during the fertile window.

Timing and understanding of your fertility are important strategies for becoming pregnant and avoiding pregnancy. It's crucial to understand that when utilized alone, they can not be as successful as other strategies. Before depending only on these techniques for family planning, couples should think carefully about their willingness to track and their comprehension of them. When it comes to time and fertility, speaking with a healthcare professional may provide specialized advice and suggestions.

How to Have a Healthy Pregnancy

For people or couples who want to establish a family, getting ready for a safe pregnancy is an essential step. A good pregnancy includes many lifestyle, health, and wellbeing factors and starts before conception. The following actions are necessary to be ready for a healthy pregnancy:

Consult a healthcare professional:
Make an appointment for a preconception checkup with a doctor who specializes in obstetrics or reproductive health.
Talk to your doctor about your pregnancy intentions, health history, family history, and any underlying issues.

Examine all of your current medicines; some may need to be altered or modified to be safe for use during pregnancy.

Vitamins for pregnancy and folic acid:
Before conception, start taking a prenatal vitamin or folic acid supplement. In the growing fetus, folic acid helps prevent neural tube abnormalities.
Start using these vitamins ideally a month or more before attempting pregnancy.

How to Reach a Healthy Weight

Keep a healthy body weight before becoming pregnant. Conditions such as being underweight or overweight may have an impact on fertility and the health of a pregnancy.
To reach and maintain a healthy weight, strive for a balanced diet and consistent exercise.

Stop using drugs, alcohol, and smoking:
Avoid using recreational drugs, drinking, or smoking before becoming pregnant since they may damage the fetus and raise pregnancy risks.

Chronic Conditions to Manage:
Work with your healthcare professional to make sure any chronic health issues, such as diabetes, hypertension, or epilepsy, are properly controlled prior to conception.
During pregnancy, several problems could call for specific treatment.

Performing an infection check

Make sure your vaccines are current since certain illnesses that may be prevented by vaccinations can be dangerous to an unborn child.

Sexually transmitted infections (STIs) should be screened for since untreated infections might cause problems during pregnancy.

Maintaining Mental Health and Stress:
High stress levels and untreated mental health issues may have an impact on a woman's ability to conceive and deliver a baby.
If necessary, use stress-reduction strategies like mindfulness, meditation, or therapy.

Limit Your Exposure to Environmental Hazards and Toxins:
Reduce exposure to dangerous substances and environmental contaminants that may damage fertility and fetal development, such as lead or pesticides.

Choices for a Healthy Lifestyle:

Adopt a healthy lifestyle that consists of consistent exercise, a well-balanced food, and enough sleep.
Avoid consuming coffee in excess, and talk to your doctor about any dietary issues.

Learn About Your Cycle and Fertility:
To determine the most viable days for conception, monitor your menstrual cycle and ovulation.
Knowing your fertility status might help you plan your pregnancy.

Emotional and Financial Preparedness:
Examine your financial preparedness for motherhood, taking into account daycare and medical bills.
Think about how emotionally prepared you are for parenthood's demands.

Goals for Family Planning:
Talk openly and honestly with your spouse about your family planning objectives, such as how many kids you want and when to have them.

Look for Assistance and Information:
To learn more about pregnancy, delivery, and parenting, join support groups or look for information from reliable sources.
You may prepare emotionally and make educated choices with the aid of education and assistance.

A proactive and crucial phase is preparing for a healthy pregnancy. It prepares the mother and the unborn child for a successful and healthy pregnancy. A good pregnancy and safe delivery are made possible by regular prenatal care, healthy lifestyle choices, and early intervention where necessary. A healthcare professional you consult with may provide you individualized advice and suggestions based on your unique health and family planning requirements.

CHAPTER FIVE

Maternity Wellness

Early Pregnancy Symptoms and Signs
The signs and symptoms of early pregnancy might differ from person to person, and some people may notice them more obviously than others. Take a home pregnancy test or speak with a healthcare professional for confirmation if you think you may be pregnant. Here are some typical pregnancy warning signs and symptoms:

Period Missed:
A missing menstrual cycle is among the most typical early indicators of pregnancy. However, minor spotting or irregular bleeding during the first trimester of pregnancy might happen to certain women.

Breast alterations
One to two weeks following pregnancy, breast enlargement and pain might start.

The areolas (the darker region around the nipples) may darken and nipples may become more sensitive.

Fatigue:
During the first few weeks of pregnancy, a lot of pregnant people feel very exhausted and worn out, often as a result of hormonal changes.

Urinating a lot:
Increased blood flow to the pelvic region brought on by hormonal changes might result in more frequent urination. As early as six to eight weeks during pregnancy, this sensation might appear.

Morning Malaise:
Beginning in the first few weeks of pregnancy, morning sickness is characterized by nausea and vomiting. Any time of day might see it.
Morning sickness is not a universal symptom of pregnancy, and its intensity might vary.

Changes in Food Cravings and Aversions:

Food desires and aversions might result from changes in taste and scent sensitivity. These may drastically differ between people.

A light abdominal cramp:
Early in pregnancy, when the uterus starts to enlarge, some pregnant people may suffer minor uterine cramps.

Mood Changes
Hormonal changes might cause mood swings, impatience, or a heightened sensitivity to emotions.
Body's normal core temperature
A persistently elevated basal body temperature (BBT) may be a sign of pregnancy for those who use it as a fertility awareness tool.

Increased Smell Sense:
Some individuals report that during the first trimester of pregnancy, their sense of smell sharpens.

Bloating and constipation:

Hormonal fluctuations might cause digestion to become sluggish and bloated.

More vaginal discharge
Leukorrhea, a rise in vaginal discharge, is a typical occurrence during pregnancy. It must be odorless and white or transparent.

Fainting or dizziness:
When rising up fast, changes in blood pressure and blood flow might cause lightheadedness or fainting.

It's crucial to remember that these symptoms may also be brought on by other illnesses or even for causes unrelated to pregnancy. Use a home pregnancy test or get confirmation from a healthcare professional if you think you may be pregnant. In order to monitor the health of both the pregnant woman and the growing baby, early prenatal care is essential, hence it is advised to seek medical guidance as soon as pregnancy is suspected.

Prenatal Care and Examinations

A healthy pregnancy must include prenatal care and routine checkups. Proper prenatal care guarantees prompt interventions when needed, offers information and support, and aids in monitoring the health of the pregnant woman and the growing baby. Here is a summary of prenatal care and examinations:

1. How Vital Prenatal Care Is:
For a healthy pregnancy and safe delivery, prenatal care must begin early and be consistent.
It lowers the chance of problems by enabling healthcare professionals to see and manage any possible health concerns early on.
Prenatal care offers chances to learn about diet, exercise, and pregnancy-related issues.
It provides the expectant mother and her spouse with emotional support and direction.

2. Beginning Prenatal Care:
The optimal time to start prenatal care is as soon as pregnancy is known to be present, usually

after a positive result from a home pregnancy test.

Make an appointment for your first prenatal visit with a healthcare professional if you think you may be pregnant.

3. Prenatal check-up frequency:
Pregnancy checkup frequency might change based on a woman's health and risk factors. A normal timetable, however, may consist of:
Weeks 1 through 12 of the first trimester include monthly checkups.
Throughout the second trimester's (weeks 13–28) bimonthly checkups
Throughout the third trimester's (weeks 29–40) weekly visits

4. Prenatal check-up components:
Physical examination: This include determining the baby's development and positioning as well as taking blood pressure, weight, and belly size measurements.
Regular urinalyses to check for protein, hyperglycemia, or infection symptoms.

Blood tests: Regular blood work to screen for infections and illnesses including gestational diabetes as well as to check for anemia, blood type, Rh factor, and other problems.

Regular ultrasounds are used to check on the baby's health, development, and location.
Heartbeat monitoring: Following the first trimester, listening to the baby's heartbeat.
Genetic testing: An optional procedure that may be explored with a healthcare professional to check for genetic abnormalities or birth problems.
Education and Counseling: Advice on healthy eating, physical activity, prenatal vitamins, and labor preparation.
Discussing emotional health, responding to worries, and offering assistance are all examples of emotional support.

5. Particularized Care:
A few pregnancies could need particular treatment because of underlying illnesses or other risky circumstances. In certain situations,

healthcare professionals may recommend additional specialists or maternal-fetal medicine experts to pregnant patients.

6. After-birth care:

Postpartum treatment continues the prenatal phase. Attending postpartum check-ups is crucial to ensuring a quick recovery and addressing any issues with breastfeeding, contraception, and postpartum health.

7. Getting in Touch With Your Healthcare Professional:

Throughout your pregnancy, it's crucial to have frank conversations with your doctor.

Any signs, discomforts, or strange alterations in your health or well-being should be discussed.

Anytime you have questions or concerns about your treatment or your pregnancy, ask them and get answers.

Regular prenatal care is linked to better results for both the mother and the unborn child. It makes it possible to identify and handle any issues early on, resulting in a healthier pregnancy and delivery. For the finest treatment throughout pregnancy, always heed the advice of your healthcare professional and go to all scheduled prenatal checkups.

Exercise and Nutrition During Pregnancy

For the health of both the pregnant woman and the growing baby, proper diet and exercise are crucial. Making healthy decisions may promote a pleasant pregnancy, lower the chance of problems, and speed up the postpartum healing process. Pregnancy diet and exercise recommendations are as follows:

Eating Well While Pregnant:

Healthy Eating:
Concentrate on eating a balanced diet that consists of a range of foods from all dietary categories, including fruits, vegetables, healthy grains, lean proteins, and dairy or dairy substitutes.

folic acid and foliate:
Make sure you are getting enough folic acid, a B vitamin that aids in protecting the developing embryo from neural tube abnormalities. Foods like leafy greens, fortified cereals, and supplements all contain it.

Iron:
More iron is required during pregnancy to sustain the larger blood volume. Lean meats, beans, lentils, and fortified cereals are good sources of iron.

Calcium:
To aid in the growth of the baby's bones and teeth, eat calcium-rich foods like leafy greens, fortified plant-based milk, and dairy products.

Protein:
Include lean meats, chicken, fish, beans, tofu, and nuts as sources of protein in your diet.

Hydration:

Stay hydrated by drinking plenty of water, particularly if you're pregnant since your body requires more fluids.

Avoid alcohol and limit caffeine:
Avoid consuming too much coffee since it may increase the risk of difficulties during pregnancy. Alcohol should be completely avoided when pregnant.
Seafood and Fish:
Whenever possible, choose low-mercury choices like salmon and shrimp when eating fish and seafood.

Fiber:
To treat constipation, a typical pregnant symptom, include high-fiber meals like whole grains, fruits, and vegetables in your diet.

Supplements:
To ensure that you are achieving your nutritional requirements, including those for folic acid and iron, take prenatal vitamins as directed by your healthcare professional.

Workout While Pregnant:

Consult a healthcare professional
Consult your doctor before beginning or maintaining an exercise program while pregnant. They may provide tailored advice depending on your state of health and fitness.

Remain Active:
Being active when pregnant is typically a good thing. Prenatal yoga, swimming, stationary cycling, and walking may all help you stay healthy and ease pain.

Safety and moderation:
Select low-impact workouts and stay away from anything that puts you at a high risk of falling or being hurt. Avoid engaging in contact sports or other activities where there is a chance of suffering an abdominal injury.

Take Note of Your Body:

During exercising, pay attention to how your body feels. Stop exercising and see your doctor if you have any discomfort, wooziness, shortness of breath, or other unsettling symptoms.

Exercises for the Pelvis:
To assist the pelvic muscles get stronger and support the developing uterus while lowering the risk of incontinence, think about doing pelvic floor exercises (Kegels).

Keep from Overheating:
Avoid overheating at all costs since it might damage the growing fetus. Drink plenty of water and work out in a room with good ventilation.

Body mechanics and posture:
To lower the risk of back pain and other pregnancy-related discomforts, keep a decent posture and employ appropriate body mechanics.

Exercises Modified:
Some workouts may need to be changed or stopped as the pregnancy goes on. For advice,

speak with a physical therapist or prenatal fitness instructor.

Rest and Restoration

To avoid overexertion, make sure you have enough rest and recuperation time in between workout sessions.

Working with your healthcare professional to develop a tailored diet and fitness plan that takes into account your particular requirements and circumstances is crucial since every pregnancy is different. The best way to encourage a healthy pregnancy and promote the wellbeing of both you and your unborn child is to be educated, make healthy decisions, and seek expert advice when necessary.

CHAPTER SIX

Pregnancy and Birth Control:
Taking Care of Birth Control While Pregnant

Several significant factors must be taken into account while using birth control when pregnant: Discontinuing Birth Control: As soon as a pregnancy is established, all forms of birth control must be abandoned. Continued use of birth control throughout pregnancy is unnecessary and may even be detrimental since pregnancy itself serves as a natural contraceptive.

Consult a healthcare professional: Once pregnancy has been confirmed, make an appointment with an obstetrician or healthcare professional to begin prenatal care. Discuss your medical history, any past use of birth control, and any pertinent health facts at this visit.

Review of Medications: The healthcare professional may go through your medication history if you previously used hormonal birth control methods, such as birth control pills. To ensure that some drugs are safe to use during pregnancy, they may need to be changed or stopped. You will get advice on any required modifications from your healthcare practitioner.

Prenatal Care: Receiving routine prenatal care should be the main priority throughout pregnancy. Healthcare professionals will keep an eye on the pregnant woman's health as well as the health of the growing baby, look for any possible difficulties, and provide advice on diet, exercise, and other components of a healthy pregnancy.

Future Family Planning: While contraception during pregnancy is not required, it is a good opportunity to talk with your healthcare professional about future family planning. They can tell you about the many postpartum contraceptive methods available and assist you in making an informed decision based on your preferences and medical needs.

Protection Against Sexually Transmitted Infections (STIs): Using condoms may provide protection if you participate in sexual activity while pregnant and are worried about STIs. Even while pregnancy itself functions as a natural contraceptive, it does not provide STI protection.

After giving delivery, you may talk with your healthcare professional about your postpartum contraceptive choices. Your unique situation, your intention to breastfeed, and your health concerns may all influence your decision on a contraceptive technique.

Nursing with Contraception:
 It's vital to think about birth control options that work with nursing if you want to breastfeed after giving delivery. While certain forms of contraception are better suited for women who are nursing, others may harm the infant or the mother's milk supply. Your healthcare practitioner may advise you on the best forms of contraception.

Keep in mind that pregnancy is a natural type of birth control, thus birth control should be stopped once pregnancy is established. To ensure a successful pregnancy and delivery, concentrate on getting complete prenatal care. Don't be afraid to talk to your healthcare practitioner if you have any queries or worries regarding birth control or family planning. They can give advice and help that is catered to your particular need.

CONCLUSION

In conclusion, birth control and pregnancy are important parts of reproductive health that affect people's lives in different ways. The birth of a new life and the accompanying physical and emotional changes make pregnancy a profoundly changing experience. Preconception health, diet, exercise, and prenatal care are just a few proactive steps that go into planning for a successful pregnancy.

Regular check-ups and appropriate medical assistance are necessary during pregnancy to safeguard the health of both the pregnant woman and the growing baby.

Contrarily, people who want to delay becoming pregnant until they are prepared for motherhood should use birth control as a crucial tool. It includes a variety of techniques, from non-hormonal ones like condoms and fertility education to hormonal ones like birth control pills and implants. The type of birth control chosen should suit the tastes, health needs, and family planning objectives of the person.

People are more equipped to make wise choices regarding family planning and contraception when they have a basic understanding of the female reproductive system, the menstrual cycle, and fertility awareness.

Additionally, selecting a birth control technique that takes into account aspects like side effects, efficacy, and personal lifestyle may result in a more positive and productive experience.

Open communication with healthcare professionals is essential at every stage of life, from conception through delivery and beyond. In order to meet specific health requirements and family planning objectives, they may provide direction, encouragement, and specialized advice.

Knowledge and making educated decisions are crucial, whether one is choosing to postpone or avoid becoming a parent or is already on the route to motherhood. Birth control and pregnancy are important chapters in the intricate and beautiful tale of life, and by approaching them with consideration and awareness, people may travel both paths with assurance and well-being.